GUT FIT –
FAT GONE

PAUL ENDERS

Contents

Preface

Let me get to the point. I have always been fat. There is no time in my past I can recall where I was not carrying too much weight.

I was fat as a child, as a teenager, and as an adult, and I know there is no age in which „being fat"doesn't have significant disadvantages. Teased as a kid, and as a teenager as well. And when the hormones started to get active – you can probably imagine.

As a grown-up I did not really get ahead in my career, and was often overtaken by less qualified people – in job interviews I lost to streamlined handsome people... It is no fun being fat. The worst thing about it – the attitude I developed; the disposition, the heavy bones, the parents growing up, the load of bad experiences in my childhood – all that was at fault. Everything but the person stuffing his face with various foods and sugary drinks: Me.

I busied myself with the mantra „I feel good just the way I am ". - had I used just one part of the energy I was wasting to convince myself and everyone else I was „feeling good" for measures to actually feel good, I would probably look different today, and my life would have gone another way.

I am not complaining. Today I know that I did all that to myself. I take responsibility for all the wasted years, harming my health, and the many unreached goals, and I am working on giving my best day after day in order to design my remaining years or decades in a more beautiful and more happy and healthy way.

Today I am almost half a quintal lighter, and on my best way to tackle the remaining kilos. Many people have approached me in the past few days and months and asked how I managed to do that, and I think in all my life I had never received as much encouragement and acknowledgement as I do now that I can fit into a clothing size you can find in any clothing store.

By now there are many people who let themselves get inspired by me and went on their way to tackle their weight problem. A dear friend of mine, Leo, has suggested that I write my experiences down in order to let other people benefit from them so they can take the same way I did.

The most exciting thing about the whole story is that I did not even notice I was dieting when I lost the weight. I had an entirely different goal at the time, and I am happy that I have reached that as well.

I realise that, as the people in Cologne use to say, „every fool is different". That could mean that my way is not your way, and that your body needs something entirely different. I cannot promise you anything, but I want to let you benefit from my experiences and my methods, so you have a basis for your decision that you should consult an expert on.

I wish you lots of success,
Paul Enders

ONE

DIET? - THAT WAS NOT PLANNED

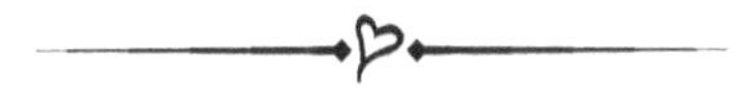

Had someone told me to start dieting, I would have indignantly refused. Of course, I had several extra kilos, or more like several dozens of them, but diets? That was not for me. I had already tried dozens of diets throughout my life and every single one of them ended with me being heavier than ever before.

I did not want to diet at any price. But I had a huge problem. Almost every day I started out „normally" (if still morbidly obese), and throughout the day I noticed my belly bloating more and more. That went so far that trousers that were 4 centimetres too wide in the morning became so tight in the evening that they were strangling me.

One could think that I was simply eating too much. That this was not true could be easily proven, as the bloated belly also came when I drank only water throughout the day. I had a problem, and the first thing I tried was a product I had seen an advertising of – it was designed to reduce the bloating. Apart from the contents of my wallet this medicine did not reduce anything though, despite my keeping to the dosage instructions.

I was desperate and I would have tried anything with the slightest chance of success.

As many other times in my life, I met a friend who excitedly told me about his successes. He told me that he had the same problem (even if at a smaller scale) but could tackle it with herbal supplements within a special dietary program.

My friend spoke only of the bowel – and in no way of dieting or losing weight – otherwise I would probably not have listened. During this talk, and after it, I have read up on a lot about the bowels, and I would like to show you what I have found:

TWO

BOWELS AND BOWEL HEALTH

Some people carry around more than ten kilos of old, dried-out feces within their intestines every day, which prevents the bowel from working at its full capacity. Most people do not like to think about their bowels. All that seems intimate, dirty, and uncomfortable to us.

You are what you eat.[1]

If we think a bit further from this old phrase, a person is not really what he eats, but which of the things eaten remain in the bowel. But if you see the bowel as a kind of interface between food intake and body, this thinking is too simple.

Our body contains a secondary nervous system centered in the bowel that is so complex that it's often called the „second brain". It contains about 500 million neurons, spans about ten metres, and is located between the oesophagus and the anus. That is the „brain" responsible for your craving sweets, crisps, or other snacks when under stress or bored.

Within the intestinal wall there is the enteric nervous system controlling the digestion. More and more studies suggest that it has a large influence on our psychological and physiological condition.

The bowel-brain is independent. It feels, and it is the centre of what we mean when we are talking about a gut feeling. It warns us from environmental hazards we cannot or hardly detect deliberately, and it influences our reactions. The bowel-brain is the oldest nervous system there is. It has been verified in vertebrates from 500 million years in the past.

Indeed, experience shows that bowel health plays a central role in the physical and psychological wellbeing of a person.

The bowel is, to make it simple, divided into the large and the small intestine. The small intestine receives the food components while the large intestine dehydrates the remaining food bolus and adding the body's waste products to it. A rule of thumb is that the intestinal contents dry up and compress more, the longer they remain in the large intestine.

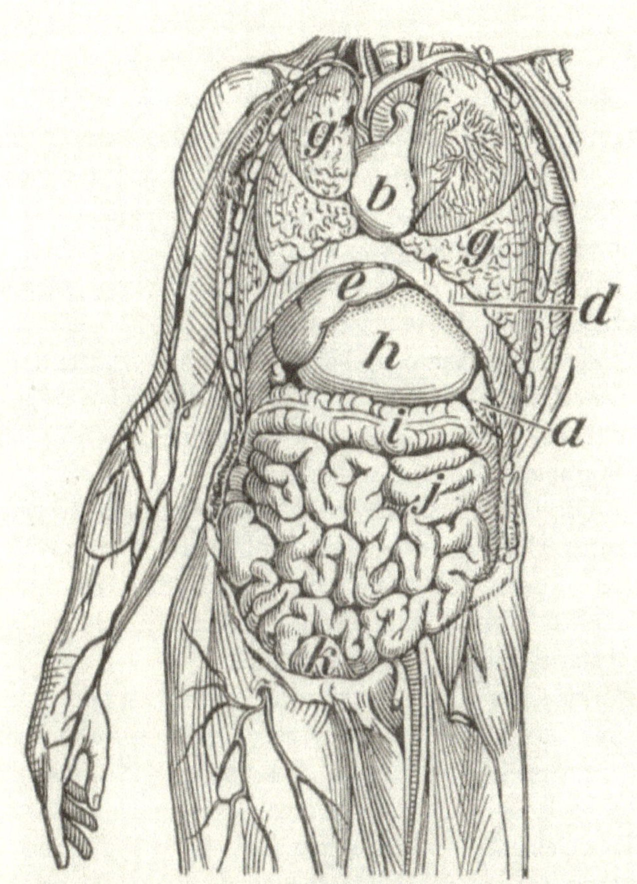

FIG. 52. — Front view of the viscera. *a*, spleen; *b*, heart; *d*, diaphragm; *e*, liver; *g*, lung; *h*, stomach; *i*, large intestine; *j* small intestine; *k*, bladder.

In a healthy bowel it has the power to transport the entire contents to the anus. Unfortunately, it is expected that most people suffer from chronic constipation. That does not necessarily mean that they do not excrete anything. Most people have bulges and pockets in their large intestine walls that have come up due to deposits. Here, dry and highly compressed intestinal contents are stored. Also, mucilage and fungus growth as well as putrifactive bacteria have taken hold of the large intestine, and it cannot excrete those on its own.

Again and again a „backlog" of these substances is created in the small intestine, which can lead to build-up on those intestinal walls as well, resulting in nutrients not being absorbed properly anymore.

Indeed this happens much more often that we would assume. But that also means that in extreme cases, a large part of good and healthy ingredients that the body is supplied with in the form of valuable foods or vital substances cannot be absorbed at all.

This leads to an effect that various market participants value very highly: The body needs more drugs and vital substances so that it can absorb anything at all. What is just as bad is that a body that realises certain vitamins and trace elements lacking reacts with hunger. This is also the reason why people who eat too much – even if they mainly eat „healthy" foods – still suffer from a deficiency in certain vital substances.

What's even more dangerous is the fact that putrefactive bacteria and fungi secrete toxins that affect the whole body. Peter Carl Simons explained that with the example of parodontids in his book „Chlorophyll – Gesundheit ist grün"[2]_

One could assume that a strong laxative could help cleansing the bowels and solving all problems. In fact, though, that is a misconception. Laxatives are based on stimulating the bowels to excrete stuff until the laxative itself has come out again.

The deposits on the intestinal walls, however, are hardly or not at all reduced or even softened. Additionally, consuming common laxatives too often may lead to a weakening of the bowels that can in many cases lead to addiction.

Reputable scientists believe that the permanent over-excitation of the bowel with laxatives will even worsen the deposits of feces in the bowel, because the over-excited bowel has less power for transportation.

The only known sustainable method for softening and excreting the deposits is intestinal cleansing. It works as a rehabilitation method for the intestine and indirectly affects health and wellbeing.

Intestinal problems

Research is just underway to recognise relations that our ancestors, and especially the old healers Galen, Hildegard von Bingen, Paracelsus or Kneipp have known for a long time. Among them:

Chronic diarrhoea

Intestinal problems can take many forms. One of the most common phenomenons is chronic diarrhoea. It can have various reasons. It seems to be the opposite of the constipation already mentioned. In truth, however, the opposite often seems to be the case:

In the slimy and crusty substances that are deposited on the intestinal wall, harmful bacteria or even intestinal parasites often cause irritations that can cause chronic diarrhoea. A multitude of worm species can find an ideal habitat within the intestine if they are full of fecal residue. They can multiply and attack the body itself. If during the intestinal cleansing the old material is excreted, usually the parasites are thrown out as well, and the irritation leading to chronic diarrhoea disappears withing a few days.

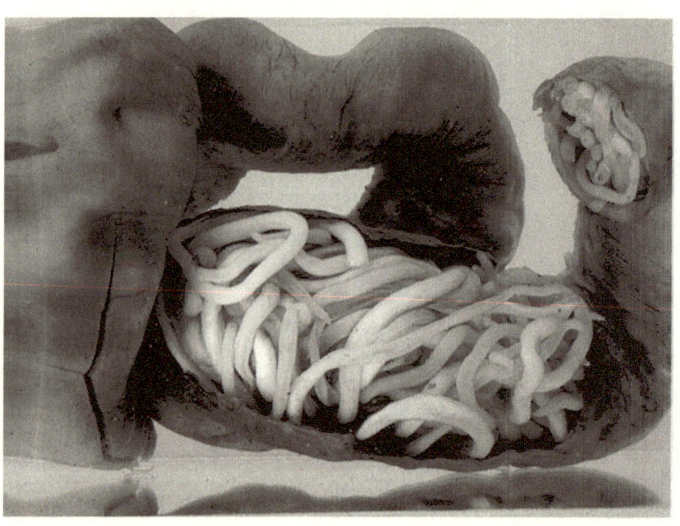

Reduced intake of nutrients

The intake (or resorption) of nutrients from the consumed foods is the main task of the intestine. This resorption capability is reduced by deposits on the intestinal wall. Most affected substances are macro molecules of proteins (amino acids), vitamins, and enzymes. This is especially maddening if someone is putting a lot of money into vitamin supplements, enzymes or trace elements, as well as protein supplements.

In many cases the initial higher consumption brings with it an improved wellbeing. Unfortunately, it will not take long, as many of these supplements (except spirulina and yeast products) have mucous generating effects. It will lead into a vicious circle. The affected person must consume more and more supplements just to hold the current level. At the same time the heightened consumption of bad protein supplements leads to an additional burden, and with it to a decrease, for the digestive functions.

Among experts it is known that even by supplementing with all known vitamins, herbal substances and trace elements in high doses, it would still end in deficiencies, because not all vital substances in our food could be identified and reproduced by far yet. This is also the reason why the only sensible way of taking in all needed substances is through the consumed food and optimising that through intestinal cleansing.

Depending on the life situation and the health condition of a person, it is important to prevent or fix deficiencies by taking in the right vital substances.

Autointoxication

If fecal residues remain in the large intestine for a long time, they start to purify. That may lead to a high concentration of harmful bacteria. Overt consumption of meat accelerates this development. The toxins secreted during this process travel throughout the body by bloodstream and reach every cell of the body. This intoxication can weaken the entire organism and lead to various diseases.

By cleansing the intestine and removing the fecal residues from the intestine, so it can function properly, prevents petrifaction. A healthy intestine excretes the contents before they can purify.

Body odour

The putrefactive processes in our intestine result in body odour. If you cannot control your body odour despite thorough hygiene, chances are that you are suffering from putrefactive activity in your large intestine.

Examples for further illnesses and injuries of the intestine that are positively affected by intestinal cleansing are hernias (diaphragmatic hernia, inguinal hernia), haemorrhoids and others.

If you intend to get deeper into the topic of intestinal health, you can have a look at the bibliography in the end. The short and partly simplified depiction of the relations in this chapter are designed to make my thoughts and processes more transparent.

Hyperacidity and intestinal health

Most authors, but also providers of intestinal cleansing programs, separate the two topics of hyperacidity and intestinal health, or at least do not explicitly formulate the necessity of tackling both topics together.

Undoubtedly, hyperacidity not only affects the intestine but also the health of the person itself.

Hyperacidity always means an attack on the intestine. Choosing an approach for intestinal cleansing that builds up the intestinal health with lots of effort, without considering the devastating effect of hyperacidity, will not reach sustainable results. Accordingly, it is important to tackle both topics at the same time if pre-existing hyperacidity is not supposed to jeopardise the intestinal cleansing.

Dr. med. Robert Bachmann states in his book „Natürlich gesund durch Säure-Basen-Gleichgewicht":

„The body must protect itself from an overt onslaught of acid. In a sense, it closes counters: The intestinal villi no longer accept acidic bolus, and promptly show it out the door. That means diarrhoea. You are familiar with it if you have eaten too much unripe fruit. This acid protection should not be prevented by fighting the diarrhoea with drugs! (...)

Within a normal, healthy microflora, there are germs important for the normal function of the large intestine, living off fibres. If the bolus reaches the large intestine, however, still containing undigested carbohydrates and proteins, it feeds germs that are specialised in these substances. They ferment the carbohydrates into acids and inferior alcohols, two substance groups vying for the place of being the most harmful to the health. "

Reproducing the whole topic group of hyperacidity and balance of acid-base-level would go far beyond the limits of this book. If you want to know more about it, you can find various interesting publications on the topic within the bibliography.

[1]Ludwig Feuerbach

[2]Simons, Peter Carl: Chlorophyll – Gesundheit ist gründ, 2015, BOD- will soon be available also in English

language

THREE

FITNESS FOR THE BOWEL

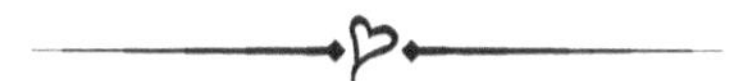

I had heard the keyword „bowel fitness" during a lecture, and I think that it describes the approach for reaching the goal well. However, you should not imagine this fitness as exotic gymnastics program. It is more about stimulating the bowel to get rid of substances that inhibit in in its functions, so that it can regain the flexibility it needs to ensure our digestion sustainably.

While I am showing you my approach, I will also list the used products and their manufacturers. This is an experience report only, and in no way advertisement or an invitation to buy and consume said products. I am convinced that there are countless good alternative products that I have not used for any of the mentioned applications, and which I can naturally not judge.

The intestinal cleansing, I did was in essence based on three components supported by one or more auxiliary agents each:

- The actual intestinal cleansing (fecal residue, fungi, putrefactive bacteria, etc.)
- The reduction of the hyperacidity
- The supply with high quality vital substances and proteins

The intestinal cleansing

It is the aim of this component to get the bowel moving, to dissolve crusts and to actively cleanse the intestine. The intestinal flora is optimised, and the immune system is strengthened by reactivating the metabolism.

Detoxication plays an especially important role in the intestine. It is its goal to remove old residue which causes illnesses, body odour, or diarrhoea through putrefaction and fungi, and to kill and excrete possible parasites.

I have used three products of the internationally active manufacturer Unicity. These are sold under the name of Unicity Cleanse, and consist of the products:

- Unicity Paraway Plus
- Unicity Lifiber
- Unicity Aloe Vera

Unicity Paraway Plus

This is a food supplement with sweeteners and, according to the packaging, the following ingredients:

Psyllium seed husk powder, guar gum, maltodextrin, fructo-oligosaccharide, apple, pectin, orange aroma, citrus pectin, hibiscus blossom powder, lifiber herbal mix 1.4%

(lucerne powder, burdock root powder, aloe vera leaf extract, cayenne pepper powder, clove powder, corn style powder, fenugreek seed powder, garlic bulb powder, ginger root powder, mallow root powder, papaya fruit extract, peppermint leaf powder, pumpkin seed powder, cranberry leaf powder), banana aroma, sweetener: sucralose, liquorice root powder, and the note that the product may contain traces of nuts.

Essentially, the product is used as a combination of active ingredients and fibres. In the context of the intestine, Wikipedia.de has the following to say about fibres:

The fibres contained within the bolus are capable of binding water, which leads to a steady increase in volume – bolus rich in fibres therefore causes additional pressure for the intestinal wall, stimulating the peristalsis, which shortens the duration fibre-rich foods remain within the intestine (as opposed to the stomach).

No higher animal has its own enzymes to break up water-insoluble fibres, especially celluloses – the ability of ruminants to break it down anyway is attributed to microorganisms living in their rumen. These microorganisms are missing in the large and small intestines, so that water-insoluble fibres pass through the digestive tract virtually unchanged.

Part of the water-soluble fibres, however, is fermented in the large intestine by the intestinal flora, which produces varying amounts of partly odourless gases like carbon dioxide, methane and hydrogen, but also short-chain fatty acids like acetate, propionate and butyrate that in contrast to medium- or long-chain fatty acids have some special characteristics (see fat digestion) and are largely reabsorbed by the large intestine mucous layer, thus contributing to feeding the mucous layer cells.

Some fibres are herbal substances that are from the ecological viewpoint designed to deter enemies, so that badly digestible fibres can generate toxic fermentation alcohols and biogenic amines harming the intestinal mucous layer and the immune system.

Along with water, fibres also bind minerals, toxins, bile acid, as well as microorganisms, that are subsequently excreted along with the feces. In the case of a balanced diet that is no problem, but in the case of separate fibre-intake it can lead to mineral deficiency in the long term.

In the context of the intestinal cleansing, this is about mobilising the intestine and excreting toxins (that, for example, were generated within the intestine through putrifactive processes).

Unicity Lifiber

Unicity Lifiber mainly focuses on detoxication. Detoxication plays an especially important role in the intestine. It is its goal to remove old residue which causes illnesses, body odour, or diarrhoea through putrefaction and fungi, and to kill and excrete possible parasites.

Unicity Paraway Plus is, according to the packaging, a food supplement with the ingredients:

Garlic powder, gelatine capsule, walnut powder, pumpkin seed powder, clove powder, sage leaf powder, beta carotene, hyssop leaf extract, fenugreek seed powder, chamomile blossom extract, black pepper powder, peppermint leaf powder, thyme leaf powder, fennel seed powder, thiamine nitrate, and may also contain traces of nuts.

The ingredient thiamine nitrate may not be so clear to some readers. The page Pharmawiki_[1] states about thiamine:

(Vitamin B1)

Thiamine (vitamin B1) is an active ingredient from the vitamin group, playing an important role for the carbohydrate metabolism and the nervous system as a co-factor to enzymes. The active form of the vitamin is called thiamine pyrophosphate. Thiamine is used for preventing and treating vitamin B1 deficiency, illnesses of the nervous cells, and as food supplements. There are hardly any side effects thanks to the broad therapeutic bandwidth it is used in. Parenteral administration may cause hypersensitivity reactions.

(...)

Thiamine plays an important role for the carbohydrate metabolism and the nervous system as a co-factor to enzymes.

It is hard to regard Lifiber and Paraway Plus separately. If you have a closer look at the ingredients, however, their effects can not so easily be separated. Both elements support one another positively, and Paraway Plus naturally also mobilises the intestine, while Lifiber on the other hand naturally also reduces crusts. That is neither surprising nor negative, as it is the point of the entire program to build up the intestinal health.

Unicity Aloe Vera

Aloe vera has been used for treating illnesses for over six thousand years, but it has also been used to maintain and rehabilitate beauty and health.

The author Peter Carl Simons compiled an impressive and easily readable portrait of this plant and its applications in his book „Aloe Vera – 6'000 Jahre Medizingeschichte können sich nicht irren: Was Ihnen die

Pharma-Industrie nicht erzählt – aber schon zu Kleopatras Zeiten jedes Kind wusste".

In the context of intestinal cleansing, the active ingredient acemannan plays a central role. Simons states:

Aloe contains a broad spectrum of carbohydrates important for our body, such as aldopentose, galactose, glucuronic acid, glucose, mannose, rhamnose, xylose and cellulose. One of the most important substances for our body is acemannan_[2]

This ingredient is regarded by many scientists as a possible active ingredient against the HI-Virus and against certain kinds of cancer. Both application areas are still being researched and are only possibilities at best. What is clear among leading scientists, however, is an improved cell respiration that in turn positively affects the entire metabolism, but also the detoxication of the body.

What is also documented is an intestinal cleansing effect combined with the build-up of a healthy intestinal flora. Therefore, nutrients can be broken down more effectively, and reabsorbed into the intestinal wall.

Through the increased cell activity, acemannan strengthens the natural immune system and results in a higher protection of the body against parasites, viruses, bacteria and fungi. This is the reason why aloe should always be part of intestinal cleansing processes.

Within the Unicity Cleanse Set, there is also Unicity Aloe Vera, a food supplement with the ingredients:

Aloe vera leaf extract, hydroxypropylcellulose capsule, separating agent: silicon dioxide. It also includes the warning that it may contain traces of nuts.

Essentially, the ingredients can be summarised in a way that makes aloe vera leaf extract the only active ingredient (in a capsule as dosage form).

Reduction of Hyperacidity

« Sour makes you happy «. This at least claims a popular saying. In truth however most people are suffering from hyperacididity.

The biggest problem of hyperacididity is the blockage of intestinal villi. Acidic basically corrodes your villi and leaves holes in them. Such a damaged intestinal mucosa cannot manufacture healthy blood anymore, which leads to serious problems. The acids blockage your intestines, putrefaction starts, and your intestinal mucosa will slowly degrade, keeping doing its important part in the blood manufacturing business.

Peter Carl Simons in his book « Chlorophyll – Gesundheit ist grün: Das grüne - ein entscheidener Gesundheitsfaktor und Energie-Lieferant« writes the following about chlorophyll in connection with hyperacidity:

It is already known that a large part of all people within our cultural sphere is suffering from hyperacidity. On one side we are consuming more and more food that leads hyperacidity in our body and on the other side fruits and vegetables do not contain the same alkaline levels like in the past decades. The abundant exhaust gases in our atmosphere lead to the well-known sour rain phenomenon, which damages and basically acidifies agricultural products.

In combination with the fact that we neglect our own fitness, which reduces excess acidity through sweating, more and more people are suffering from higher and higher levels of acidity.

Chlorophyll has a positive effect on the balance alkaline-acid-balance in our bodies. To get the best effects most experts recommend taking the recommended dosage in equal parts throughout the day.

During my treating I have taken Unicity Super Green. Basically, it is just pure chlorophyll-

In fact, chlorophyll has several very positive effects on our bodies. The Swiss "Vereinigung für Vegetarismus" writes on its pages:[5]

First, chlorophyll has a balancing effect on the alkaline-acid-levels in our bodies. Certain parts of our bodies need to be more alkaline. If we have a pH scale from 1 to 14, then 7 is neutral. The blood however needs a pH level of around 7.43 to 7.45. Levels above or below represent significant danger to our bodies. There is little tolerance for imbalances. The body tries to fight an imbalance with alkaline (like calcium) or acidic minerals. In most cases alkaline minerals are needed. The body takes these from teeth. Plaque, caries and parodontids are the following consequences. The body takes the needed elements from the bones too. This leads to osteoporosis. The body starts to decompose itself to sustain its main task – living.

The chemical composition of chlorophyll is nearly identical to haemoglobin. Haemoglobin is the red pigment in the blood. The big difference is that the central core of chlorophyll consists of magnesium while haemoglobin uses trivalent iron. Iron however is present in chlorophyll too and can be exchanged very quickly with magnesium. What is the result of this change? It is blood. The leaf green is in fact forming blood.

It is surely possible to say that chlorophyll like most of the other used ingredients have a positive effect on your intestines and even whole body which during an intestinal cleansing is a welcome side-effect. Hyperacidity affects the whole body and therefore addressing and fighting problem has a positive effect on your body.

Vital Substances and Proteins

A proper supply of plant-based proteins is a core topic for complex bodily processes like for example an intestinal cleansing. Notable experts recommend a daily intake of 2g of protein per kilogram of bodyweight and day. For an adult male weighing 80kg this would add up to 80-160g of protein per day. Protein here does not only have a sustaining effect, but it is a core element of each individual cell in your body. Especially because we are trying to change our body on a cellular level through changing our habits, it is essential to supply your body with the much-needed components for this change.

Vitamins, minerals, and micronutrients, of course, are extremely important too. Ever since I read that people of our cultural sphere are suffering from nutrient deficiencies and which effects this has, I have become especially alert regarding these topics.

You could picture it likes this: A builder who has all the needed materials but no mortar to put everything together. Everything grinds to a halt. If this happens in your body, it is easy to imagine what will happen if these deficiencies continue. Further I have noticed that the daily recommended dosages on food should be understood as minimum. So if it mentions that a certain amount covers 20% of your daily need; it should be read as 20% of the minimum daily dosage to not become sick if you do not meet it over a long period of time.

Our body knows this too and craves food if it needs to cover these deficiencies. In fact, I have not had binge eating attacks since I have started to take proteins and vital substances on a regular basis. (even after the cleansing)

I have used Unicity Complete Vanilla. According to the label it contains the following ingredients:

- Energy 156 kcal / 656 kJ
- Proteins 20 g
- Carbohydrates 8 g
- Fat 4 g
- Fibres 4 g
- Sodium 0,26 g
- Vitamin A 1.500 µg-RE
- Vitamin B1 1,5 mg
- Vitamin B2 1,7 mg
- Vitamin B6 0.6 mg (46%*)
- Pantothenacid 2,4 mg (40%*)
- Folic acid 400 µg
- Niacin 20 mg-NE
- Vitamin B12 6 µg
- Vitamin C 60 mg
- Vitamin D3 10 µg
- Vitamin E 60 mg α-TE
- Biotin 300 µg
- Calcium 350 mg
- Iron 18 mg
- Magnesium 140 mg
- Zinc 15 mg
- Copper 2mg
- Mangane 2 mg
- Chrome 120 µg
- Calium 320 mg

- Iodine 173 µg

[1]Http://www.pharmawiki.ch/

[2]α (TNF-α) and interleukins (IL-1); therefore, it might help to prevent or abrogate viral infection. These three cytokines are known to cause inflammation, and interferon is released in response to viral infections. In vitro studies have shown acemannan to inhibit HIV replication; however, in vivo studies have been inconclusive.

Acemannan is currently being used for treatment and clinical management of fibrosarcoma in dogs and cats. Administration of acemannan has been shown to increase tumor necrosis and prolonged host survival; the animals have demonstrated lymphoid infiltration and encapsulation."

5http://www.vegetarismus.ch/heft/2011-4/chlorophyll.htm

FOUR

LOSING WEIGHTS HAPPENS NATURALLY

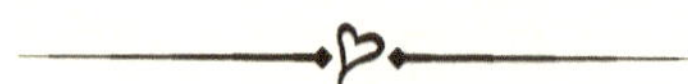

Like I already stated before, I have not started the intestinal cleansing with the goal to lose weight. This had the advantage that I was not bent on losing weight. In fact, I did not notice that I lost weight until a few days had passed and my pants were quite a bit looser than I was used too. Then of course I started monitoring the change a bit more closely.

Over the 30 days of the intestinal cleansing I have lost about 12kg and in the following time, maybe caused through a better working intestinal tract or a different way of handling nutrition, another 30kg. Especially for myself too: In the evening I do not feel as bloated as before and sleep much better. Summarised: I have completely accomplished my goal.

FIVE

MY PROGRAM

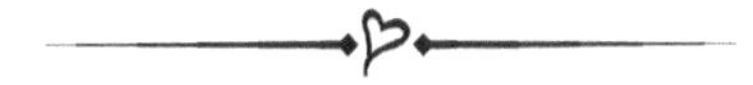

The success of this program is based on the consumed products on one side and a change in my diet on the other. It is especially important to not eat anything between the meals. Water is ok, but you should not eat or drink anything else. Alone this abdication from "eating in-between" has a positive effect on your body weight if you can endure the 30 days of the program. My regimen was the following:

Used Products

In the morning

- Unicity Paraway Plus: from the 1st-10th day; daily one capsule before breakfast; from the 11th-30th day 2 capsules after breakfast.
- Unicity Lifiber: about half an hour after Paraway Plus daily 1 measuring spoon dissolved in 250ml water; shake well and drink immediately.

- Unicity Complete Vanilla: 2 flattened measuring cups in dissolved 0.4-0.5L water or natural yoghurt as breakfast.

Midday

No special products. If you want you can eat another serving of Unicity Complete Vanilla as a shake instead of a regular meal.

Evening

Unicity Aloe Vera: from the 1st -10th day; daily one capsule for dinner; from the 11th-30th day 2 capsules for dinner.

During the day

Dissolve one measuring spoon of Unicity Super Green in 2L of water and drink the mixture evenly throughout the day.

Diet Changes

If you want to cleanse your intestines it is important to lessen the strain put on them and not give the fungi and putrefactive bacteria any more support through additional nutrients useful to them. Due to this reason a slight diet change is called for. As this program only takes 30 days these changes should be possible and endurable for anyone, especially if you are suffering from your present condition already.

Nutrition always includes beverages. To avoid increasing the acidity in your body try to abdicate from any sweet, sparkling or coffee beverages.

Breakfast

Aside from the already mentioned products (esp. Unity Complete) you do not eat anything. The nutrients in this product prevented me from feeling hungry. I felt quite energized.

Lunch

For lunch you should eat a small serving. Fill your plate until half full and do not eat any carbohydrates. Many vegetables, fruits and others contain carbohydrates, these are allowed though. Do not eat any additional ones from baked goods, rice, potatoes, bread, sugar and starch though. You should mainly eat lean meat (or fish), vegetables and salad. Vegetarians may use alternative products instead of meat that contain a high percentage of protein. Please be reminded that many of these substitution products contain a high amount of carbohydrates. Please refrain from those.

Dinner

Everything from the lunch section applies here.

In between

Abstain from any snacks and small treats between your meals. After every meal you should not at anything else for at least 4 hours (and only drink water without carbonic acid).

SIX
EPILOGUE

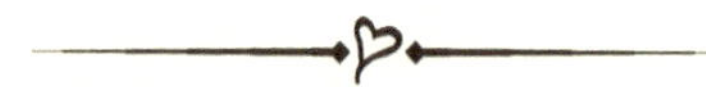

I am not a nutrition expert, doctor or schooled in medicine in any form. All my statements are my personal opinions and experiences or garnered from extensive research. This means of course that I am not offering any medical advice. For this please consult with one of the many trained experts. With my book I simply want to inspire you. Please consult with experts in the field to find out, whether the method I have presented in this book is suitable for you.

I wish you all the best and of course the required courage to be honest with yourself.

Yours,

Paul Enders

SEVEN

PRODUCT SOURCES

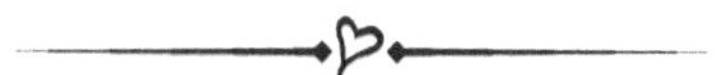

The introduced Unicity Products can be bought from local Unicity Partners.

EIGHT
LITERATURE

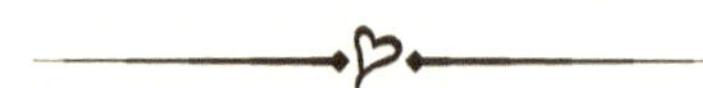

- Auer, Dr. med. W.: Übersäuerung - die stille Gefahr, 2002, Kneipp-Verlag
- Bachmann, Dr. med. R. M.: Natürlich gesund durch Säure-Basen-Gleichgewicht. Mit ihrem persönlichen 7-Tage-Programm zur sanften Entsäuerung, 2001, Trias, 2. Auflage
- Bankhofer, Prof. H.: Aloe Vera - Die Pflanze für Gesundheit, Vitalität und Wohlbefinden, 2013, Kneipp Verlag, 6. Auflage
- Dahlke, R.: Fasten Sie sich gesund - Das ganzheitliche Fastenprogramm, 2004, Irisana
- Dahlke, R., Ehrenberger, D.: Wege der Reinigung - Entgiften, entschlacken, loslassen, 2002, Heyne, 2. Auflage
- Enders, J.: Darm mit Charme, 2014, Ullstein
- Frauwallner, A.: Was tun, wenn der Darm streikt? - Probiotika sinnvoll einsetzen, 2012, Kneipp-Verlag
- Kraske, Dr. med. Eva-Maria: Säure-Basen-Balance, 2008, Gräfe und Unzer, 5. Auflage

- Lohmann, M.: Der Basen-Doktor. Basische Ernährung: gezielte Hilfe bei den häufigsten Beschwerden, 2013, Trias, 2. vollst. überarb. Auflage
- Gill, T.: Lieber schlank als sauer - Gesund ins Gleichgewicht mit der Säure-Basen-Diät, 2012, Amazon Distribution
- Gray, R.: Das Darmheilungsbuch - Gesundheit durch Kolon-Sanierung, 2011, Trias
- Jester, F.: Arginin, OPS und Entsäuerung - Power-Nährstoffe und Methoden für ein langes und gesundes Leben, 2013, Selbstverlag
- Opitz, Ch.: Befreite Ernährung - Wie der Körper uns zeigt, welche Nahrung er wirklich für Gesundheit und Wohlbefinden braucht, 2013, Hans-Nietsch-Verlag, 5. Auflage
- Schneider, G. W.: Biotop Mensch - Liebe Deine Darmbakterien, 2014, Biotop Mensch, 7. Auflage
- Thust, Th. M., Schlett, Dr. med. S.: Entgiften & entschlacken, 2006, Gräfe und Unzer
- Treutwein, N.: Übersäuerung - krank ohne Grund?, 2005, Weltbild
- Vollmer, J.B.: Gesunder Darm, gesundes Leben, 2010, Knaur
- Wacker, S., Wacker, Dr. med. A.: 300 Fragen zur Säure-Basen-Balance, 2013, Gräfe und Unzer, 2. Auflage

Disclaimer

Introduction

By using this book, you accept this disclaimer in full.

No advice

The book contains information. The information is not advice and should not be treated as such.

No representations or warranties

To the maximum extent permitted by applicable law and subject to section below, we exclude all representations, warranties, undertakings and guarantees relating to the book.

Without prejudice to the generality of the foregoing paragraph, we do not represent, warrant, undertake or guarantee:

- that the information in the book is correct, accurate, complete or non-misleading.

- that the use of the guidance in the book will lead to any particular outcome or result.

Limitations and exclusions of liability

The limitations and exclusions of liability set out in this section and elsewhere in this disclaimer: are subject to section 6 below; and govern all liabilities arising under the disclaimer or in relation to the book, including liabilities arising in contract, in tort (including negligence) and for breach of statutory duty.

We will not be liable to you in respect of any losses arising out of any event or events beyond our reasonable control.

We will not be liable to you in respect of any business losses, including without limitation loss of or damage to profits, income, revenue, use, production, anticipated savings, business, contracts, commercial opportunities or goodwill.

We will not be liable to you in respect of any loss or corruption of any data, database or software.

We will not be liable to you in respect of any special, indirect or consequential loss or damage.

Exceptions

Nothing in this disclaimer shall: limit or exclude our liability for death or personal injury resulting from negligence; limit or exclude our liability for fraud or fraudulent misrepresentation; limit any of our liabilities in any way that is not permitted under applicable law; or exclude any of our liabilities that may not be excluded under applicable law.

Severability

If a section of this disclaimer is determined by any court or other competent authority to be unlawful and/ or unenforceable, the other sections of this disclaimer continue in effect.

If any unlawful and/or unenforceable section would be lawful or enforceable if part of it were deleted, that part will be deemed to be deleted, and the rest of the section will continue in effect.

Law and jurisdiction

This disclaimer will be governed by and construed in accordance with Swiss law, and any disputes relating to this disclaimer will be subject to the exclusive jurisdiction of the courts of Switzerland.